# GLORIOUSTINA ESSIA

## Little Sprouts

### *A Family's Guide to Herbal Care for Children*

# Contents

# INTRODUCTION

## Embracing Herbal Wisdom for Your Family

Herbal care is more than just using plants to address health concerns; it's about embracing a holistic approach to wellness that considers our children's physical, emotional, and spiritual well-being. Integrating herbal remedies into our family's lives provides natural solutions for common ailments and fosters a deep connection with the natural world. This connection can instill in our children a sense of respect and appreciation for the environment and an understanding of the interconnectedness of all living things.

Herbs have been used for centuries to support health and healing, and their gentle nature makes them particularly well-suited for children's delicate systems. From soothing chamomile tea for a restful night's sleep to the immune-boosting properties of elderberry, herbs offer many benefits that can support our children's health in a gentle, nurturing way.

## The Importance of Herbal Care in Childhood

The early years of a child's life are formative in many ways, laying the foundation for their future health and well-being. Incorporating herbal care into childhood is not only about addressing immediate health concerns but also about instilling healthy habits that can last a lifetime. By choosing natural remedies, we teach our children the value of seeking gentle, non-invasive options for maintaining their health, encouraging them to listen to their bodies and to respect nature's healing power.

Moreover, herbal childhood care can help build a robust immune system, support healthy growth and development, and provide natural solutions for common childhood challenges such as teething, colic, and skin irritations. It's about empowering parents and caregivers with the knowledge and tools to care for their children in a way aligned with nature's rhythms, promoting a sense of harmony and balance that extends beyond physical health to encompass emotional and spiritual well-being.

# CHAPTER 1: FOUNDATIONS OF HERBAL CARE FOR CHILDREN

Embarking on the journey of herbal care for children requires a foundation built on understanding, safety, and guidance. This chapter aims to equip parents and caregivers with the essential knowledge needed to navigate the world of herbal remedies with confidence, ensuring that the natural solutions provided are both practical and safe for the little ones in their care.

## Understanding Children's Unique Needs

Children are not simply small adults; their bodies and systems are still developing, making their needs and responses to treatments unique. Their digestive systems, liver function, and immune systems are more delicate, requiring a gentler approach to herbal remedies. It's crucial to recognize that children's bodies process and react to herbs differently, which means dosages and formulations must be adjusted accordingly. Understanding these differences is the first step in providing effective and safe herbal care.

## Choosing Safe Herbs for Children

When it comes to selecting herbs for children, safety is paramount. Not all herbs suit young bodies; some can be harmful if misused. Here are some guidelines for choosing safe herbs for children:

- **Start with Gentle Herbs:** Opt for herbs known for their gentle, soothing properties, such as Chamomile, Lavender, and Lemon Balm. These herbs are generally well-tolerated by children and can be used for various common ailments.
- **Consult Reliable Sources:** Seek information from reputable sources, such as trusted herbalists, pediatricians with knowledge in herbal medicine, or authoritative books and websites on herbal care for children.
- **Be Aware of Allergies:** Always consider potential allergies and sensitivities. Introduce new herbs one at a time and watch for any adverse reactions.
- **Avoid Potent Herbs:** Steer clear of herbs that are known to be potent or have strong effects, such as Wormwood or Lobelia, unless under the guidance of a qualified healthcare practitioner.

## The Role of Parents in Herbal Remedies

Parents play a crucial role in their children's herbal care journey. Beyond simply administering remedies, parents are the observers, the comforters, and the decision-makers. Here's how parents can actively participate in their children's herbal care:

- **Education:** Arm yourself with knowledge about the herbs you plan to use, their benefits, and their proper application.
- **Observation:** Keep a close eye on your child's response to herbal remedies, noting any positive effects or signs of discomfort.
- **Communication:** Engage in open dialogue with your child about how they're feeling and what they're experiencing with the herbal treatments.
- **Collaboration:** Work closely with healthcare professionals, especially when dealing with more severe health issues or combining herbal and conventional therapies.

Laying the foundation for herbal care in children involves:

- A deep understanding of their unique needs.

- Careful selection of safe herbs.
- An active, informed role by parents in the application of herbal remedies.

By approaching herbal care with mindfulness and informed caution, parents can harness the gentle power of nature to support their children's health and well-being.

# CHAPTER 2: SAFE HERBS FOR CHILDREN

Introducing herbs into a child's wellness routine can be a gentle and effective way to support their health, but focusing on safety and suitability is crucial.

## Gentle Herbs for Everyday Wellness

When choosing herbs for children, starting with those known for their gentle, nurturing properties is essential.  Here are some safe and commonly used herbs for children's everyday wellness:

- **Chamomile (Matricaria recutita):** Renowned for its calming and soothing effects, Chamomile is ideal for relieving restlessness, aiding sleep, and soothing digestive upsets.
- **Lemon Balm (Melissa officinalis):** With its mild sedative properties, Lemon Balm can help reduce anxiety and promote a sense of calm in children.
- **Echinacea (Echinacea spp.):** Known for its immune-boosting properties, Echinacea can support the immune system, especially during cold and flu season.
- **Calendula (Calendula officinalis):** Gentle and soothing, Calendula is excellent for skin irritations, minor wounds, and rashes.
- **Lavender (Lavandula angustifolia):** Lavender's relaxing aroma makes it perfect for promoting relaxation and aiding sleep through direct inhalation or a calming bath.

# Dosage Guidelines for Young Bodies

Determining the correct dosage of herbs for children is crucial for their safety and efficacy. Here are some general guidelines to consider:

- **Consult a Professional:** Always consult with a healthcare professional or a qualified herbalist to determine the appropriate dosage for your child's age, weight, and health condition.
- **Start Low, Go Slow:** Begin with the lowest recommended dose and observe your child's response. You can gradually increase the dosage but always stay within the recommended range.
- **Follow Age-Appropriate Guidelines:** Dosages are often calculated based on the child's weight or age. Generally, a child's dose is typically one-third to one-half of an adult's dose.
- **Use Simple Preparations:** Opt for teas, glycerites, or mild tinctures, as these forms are more accessible for children's bodies to assimilate.

# Creating a Kid-Friendly Herbal Pantry

Having a selection of safe, child-friendly herbs can empower you to address everyday health concerns naturally. Here's how to create a kid-friendly herbal pantry:

- **Stock Up on Basics:** Include a variety of gentle herbs like Chamomile, Lemon Balm, Echinacea, and Calendula in your pantry.
- **Choose Suitable Forms:** Opt for herbal teas, glycerin-based tinctures, and gentle topical preparations that are easy for children to use.
- **Label Clearly:** Ensure all herbs and remedies are labelled with their names, dosages, and expiration dates.
- **Store Safely:** Keep your herbal pantry out of reach of children and in a cool, dry place to preserve the potency of the herbs.

# CHAPTER 3: HERBAL REMEDIES FOR COMMON CHILDHOOD AILMENTS

Children are naturally curious and active, which often leads to childhood's everyday bumps, bruises, and sniffles.

## Natural Solutions for Colds and Flu

When cold and flu season strikes, herbs can offer immune support and symptom relief:

- **Elderberry (Sambucus nigra):** Renowned for its antiviral properties, Elderberry syrup can be given at the first sign of a cold or flu to help reduce the duration and severity of symptoms.
- **Echinacea (Echinacea spp.):** This immune-boosting herb can be taken as a tea or tincture to help strengthen the body's natural defences against cold and flu viruses.
- **Ginger (Zingiber officinale):** A warm Ginger tea can help soothe sore throats, reduce fever, and alleviate nausea.

## Easing Tummy Troubles with Herbs

Digestive issues are common in children, but herbs can offer gentle relief:

- **Chamomile (Matricaria recutita):** A mild tea made from Chamomile flowers can help calm upset stomachs, reduce gas, and ease colic in infants.

- **Fennel (Foeniculum vulgare):** Fennel tea relieves indigestion and bloating, making it a go-to remedy for tummy aches.
- **Peppermint (Mentha piperita):** A soothing Peppermint tea can help relax the digestive tract, easing cramps and nausea.

## Herbal Care for Scrapes and Bruises

For the inevitable scrapes and bruises of childhood, herbs can provide natural first aid:

- **Calendula (Calendula officinalis):** Apply Calendula-infused oil or cream to minor cuts and scrapes to promote healing and prevent infection.
- **Arnica (Arnica montana):** Arnica gel or cream reduces swelling and bruising when applied topically to the affected area (avoid broken skin).

## Soothing Natural Remedies for Skin Irritations

Children's delicate skin can be prone to irritations, but herbs offer soothing solutions:

- **Aloe Vera (Aloe barbadensis):** The gel from Aloe Vera leaves can be applied directly to sunburns, rashes, or insect bites to soothe and heal the skin.
- **Oatmeal (Avena sativa):** An oatmeal bath can relieve itchy skin conditions like eczema or chickenpox. Add ground oatmeal to a warm bath and let your child soak for 15-20 minutes.

Herbal remedies provide a natural and gentle way to address common childhood ailments, from colds and flu to tummy troubles and skin irritations.

# CHAPTER 4: BUILDING IMMUNITY IN CHILDREN WITH HERBS

A robust immune system is the cornerstone of good health, especially for growing children exposed to germs and viruses.

## Strengthening Young Immune Systems Naturally

Children's immune systems are continuously developing, and certain herbs can provide gentle support during this crucial time:

- **Astragalus (Astragalus membranaceus):** This adaptogenic herb is known for its immune-boosting properties. Adding Astragalus to soups or broths can help enhance your child's natural defences.
- **Elderberry (Sambucus nigra):** Rich in antioxidants, Elderberry is excellent for supporting the immune system and can be given as a tasty syrup that children love.
- **Echinacea (Echinacea spp.):** Echinacea is well-regarded for its immune-stimulating effects. A mild Echinacea tea or tincture can be used during cold and flu season to help prevent illness.

## Preventative Herbal Tonics and Teas

Incorporating herbal tonics and teas into your child's daily routine can provide ongoing immune support:

- **Daily Immune-Boosting Tea:** Combine immune-supportive herbs like Lemon Balm, Nettle, and Rosehips. Serve this tea chilled or warm daily to keep their immune system strong.
- **Herbal Multivitamin Syrup:** Combine herbs high in vitamins and minerals, such as Nettle, Alfalfa, and Dandelion, in a syrup form. This can serve as a natural multivitamin to support overall health and immunity.

## Seasonal Herbs for Enhanced Resistance

Adapting your child's herbal regimen to the seasons can help them stay resilient throughout the year:

- **Spring and Summer:** Focus on cooling and detoxifying herbs like Dandelion and Burdock to support the liver and cleanse the blood, which supports the immune system.
- **Fall and Winter:** Shift to warming and immune-strengthening herbs like Ginger, Thyme, and Elderberry to help protect against colds and flu.

Building immunity in children with herbs is a gentle and practical approach to fostering robust health. Incorporating immune-supportive herbs into their daily routine can help your child develop a robust defence immune system against illness.

# CHAPTER 5: HERBS FOR CONCENTRATION AND CALMNESS

Herbs offer a gentle, natural way to support concentration and calmness in children, enhancing their ability to focus, learn, and relax. Incorporating herbs into their daily routine can help your child achieve a balanced state of mind and body. This chapter explores how herbs can be a gentle ally in supporting focus, learning, and relaxation, helping children navigate their days with a balanced and peaceful demeanor.

## Supporting Focus and Learning with Herbal Aids

Herbs can play a supportive role in enhancing cognitive function and attention in children:

- **Gotu Kola (Centella Asiatica):** Renowned for its cognitive-enhancing properties, Gotu Kola can support memory, concentration, and overall brain health. A mild tea or tincture can be a great addition to your child's routine during school days.
- **Lemon Balm (Melissa officinalis):** With its calming yet uplifting effects, Lemon Balm can help soothe anxiety while promoting focus and a positive mood. It's excellent for children who experience nervousness or restlessness during learning activities.
- **Ginkgo Biloba:** Known for improving circulation and cognitive function, Ginkgo can be a helpful herb for older children and adolescents to enhance

focus and mental clarity.

## Calming Herbs for Restful Sleep and Relaxation

A good night's sleep is essential for a child's health and well-being. Certain herbs can help promote relaxation and ease the transition to sleep:

- **Chamomile (Matricaria recutita):** A gentle, soothing herb, Chamomile is ideal for children, helping to calm nerves and induce a peaceful sleep. A warm cup of Chamomile tea before bedtime can become a comforting nighttime ritual.
- **Lavender (Lavandula angustifolia):** The aroma of Lavender has a calming effect on the nervous system. Incorporating Lavender oil in a bedtime bath or using a Lavender sachet under the pillow can help create a serene sleep environment.

## Balancing Energy Levels in Active Children

While energy and enthusiasm are natural in children, finding balance is crucial to their overall well-being:

- **Ashwagandha (Withania somnifera):** An adaptogenic herb, Ashwagandha can help modulate energy levels, reducing hyperactivity while boosting vitality when needed. It's best used under the guidance of a healthcare professional, especially for children.
- **Rhodiola (Rhodiola rosea):** Another adaptogen, Rhodiola, can support stamina and endurance while helping the body adapt to stress. It can benefit active children who need to sustain their energy throughout the day.

As with all herbal remedies, it's essential to consult with a healthcare professional to ensure they are appropriate and safe for your child's specific needs.

# CHAPTER 6: NUTRITIONAL HERBS FOR GROWING BODIES

Proper nutrition is a cornerstone of healthy development in children. As they grow and explore the world, their bodies require diverse nutrients to support their physical and mental well-being. This chapter delves into how nutritional herbs and superfoods can complement a child's diet, providing essential vitamins, minerals, and other beneficial compounds. By incorporating nutritional herbs and superfoods into their diets, you can support the healthy growth and development of children's bodies. These natural additions can enhance the nutritional value of meals, support digestion, and ensure that growing bodies receive the vital nutrients they need.

## Superfoods and Herbs for Nutritional Support

Incorporating nutrient-dense herbs and superfoods into a child's diet can provide a natural boost to their overall nutrition:

- **Nettle (Urtica dioica):** Rich in vitamins A, C, and K, as well as minerals like calcium and iron, Nettle is a powerful nutritional herb. It can be used in soups, teas, or smoothies to enhance a child's nutrient intake.
- **Spirulina:** This blue-green algae is packed with protein, vitamins, and minerals, making it an excellent superfood for growing bodies. It can be easily added to smoothies or yogurt for a nutritional boost.
- **Alfalfa (Medicago sativa):** Known as the "father of all foods," Alfalfa is

high in vitamins and minerals, including vitamin K, essential for bone health. It can be used in salads, sandwiches, or as a tea.

## Integrating Herbs into Child-Friendly Meals

Making herbal nutrition a part of everyday meals can be both fun and beneficial:

- **Herbal Pesto:** Blend fresh herbs like Basil, Parsley, or Cilantro with nuts, garlic, and olive oil to create a delicious pesto that can be added to pasta, sandwiches, or dip.
- **Herb-Infused Smoothies:** Add mild, nutritional herbs like Nettle or Alfalfa to fruit smoothies for an extra nutrient kick.
- **Herbal Sprinkles:** Dry and grind herbs like Dandelion leaves or Kale to make a nutrient-rich powder that can be sprinkled over meals like a seasoning.

## Herbs for Healthy Digestion and Absorption

Ensuring that children absorb the nutrients from their food is just as important as the food itself:

- **Fennel (Foeniculum vulgare):** Fennel seeds can be chewed or brewed into a tea to aid digestion and reduce gas, making it easier for children to absorb nutrients from their meals.
- **Ginger (Zingiber officinale):** A small amount can stimulate digestion and improve nutrient absorption, especially when added to meals with proteins or complex carbohydrates.
- **Peppermint (Mentha piperita):** Peppermint tea can soothe the digestive tract, reducing discomfort and improving the digestion of meals.

# CHAPTER 7: CRAFTING HERBAL REMEDIES AT HOME

Encouraging families to craft herbal remedies enriches their knowledge and bond with the natural world. This hands-on approach to managing minor health concerns and enhancing well-being can be enjoyable and instructive for all ages. Crafting herbal remedies at home provides a beautiful opportunity for families to explore the world of herbal medicine together. This chapter explores simple, safe, practical recipes and engaging projects that the whole family can enjoy.

## Simple Recipes for Children's Herbal Remedies

Here are a few easy-to-make herbal remedies that can be used for common childhood concerns:

- **Calming Chamomile Tea:** For restlessness or trouble sleeping, steep 1 teaspoon of dried Chamomile flowers in 1 cup of hot water for 10 minutes. Strain and sweeten with honey if desired. Serve warm before bedtime.
- **Lavender Sleep Spray:** Mix 10 drops of Lavender essential oil with 1 cup of water in a spray bottle. Shake well and spritz around the child's bedroom or on their pillow to promote relaxation and sleep.
- **Ginger Tummy Syrup:** Simmer a few slices of fresh Ginger root in 1 cup of water for 20 minutes. Strain and mix the liquid with an equal amount of honey. Store in the refrigerator and give 1 teaspoon for nausea or upset

stomach.

## Creating Herbal Baths, Oils, and Poultices

Herbal baths and topical applications can provide soothing relief for various conditions:

- **Herbal Bath Soak:** For a relaxing bath, tie a handful of calming herbs like Lavender, Chamomile, and Calendula in a cloth bag. Place the bag in the bathwater, allowing the herbs to infuse and create a soothing soak.
- **Calendula Infused Oil:** Gently heat dried Calendula petals in a carrier oil (like almond or olive oil) on low heat for 2-3 hours. Strain and store the infused oil in a dark bottle. Use it to soothe dry skin, rashes, or minor cuts.
- **Aloe Vera and Lavender Poultice:** Mix fresh Aloe Vera gel with a few drops of Lavender essential oil. Apply the mixture to a clean cloth and place it on sunburned or irritated skin for cooling relief.

## Fun Herbal Projects for Families

Engaging in herbal projects together can be a delightful way to learn about herbs and their uses:

- **Herb Garden:** Start a small herb garden with easy-to-grow herbs like Mint, Basil, and Parsley. Children can help with planting, watering, and harvesting, learning about each herb's properties.
- **Herbal Playdough:** Make playdough infused with child-safe essential oils like Orange or Lavender. Mix 2 cups of flour, 1 cup of salt, 2 tablespoons of oil, and 1 cup of warm water with a few drops of essential oil. Knead until smooth and enjoy the aromatic playtime.
- **DIY Herbal Lip Balm:** Melt 2 tablespoons of beeswax with 2 tablespoons of infused herbal oil (like Calendula or Chamomile) and a teaspoon of honey. Pour the mixture into small containers and let it cool. Children can use the lip balm for chapped lips or as a natural balm for minor scrapes.

By involving children in these activities, you teach them valuable skills and instill a lifelong appreciation for the healing power of plants.

# CHAPTER 8: INTEGRATING HERBAL PRACTICES INTO DAILY LIFE

Incorporating herbal practices into daily life can transform how families approach health and wellness. It's about more than just remedies; it's about cultivating a lifestyle that honors the healing power of plants. This chapter explores practical ways to make herbs seamless in family routines, educate children about herbal wisdom, and grow a family herb garden.

## Making Herbs a Part of Family Routines

Incorporating herbs into daily routines can be simple and enjoyable:

- **Herbal Teas:** Start the day or wind down in the evening with a family tea time. Choose teas that suit the time of day, such as energizing Mint in the morning or calming Chamomile at night.
- **Cooking with Herbs:** Encourage children to add fresh or dried herbs to meals. Discuss the flavors and health benefits of each herb as you cook together.
- **Herbal Self-Care:** Introduce herbal products into your family's self-care routines, such as using herbal toothpaste, soaps, or shampoos. This can be a gentle way to integrate the benefits of herbs into everyday life.

# Teaching Children About Herbal Wisdom

Educating children about herbs can foster a deep respect for nature and its healing gifts:

- **Herb Identification:** Take walks in nature and teach children to identify local herbs. Discuss their traditional uses and how they can be used safely.
- **Storytelling:** Share stories or folklore about herbs and their magical properties. This can spark children's imagination and interest in herbal medicine.
- **Simple Remedies:** Involve children in making simple herbal remedies, such as a Lavender sachet for their pillow or a Calendula salve for minor scrapes. This hands-on experience can be both educational and empowering.

# Cultivating a Family Herb Garden

Growing an herb garden is a rewarding way for families to connect with nature:

- **Planning Together:** Let each family member choose a few herbs they want to grow. Research their needs and plan the garden layout together.
- **Planting and Caring:** Involve children in planting and assign them tasks like watering or weeding. This helps them learn about plant care and responsibility.
- **Harvesting and Using:** When the herbs are ready, harvest them together and use them in meals, teas, or remedies. This full-circle experience can deepen the family's appreciation for herbs.

Integrating herbal practices into daily life is a journey that can bring families closer to nature and each other. Making herbs part of family routines, teaching children about herbal wisdom, and cultivating a family herb garden can create a holistic lifestyle that nurtures the body, mind, and spirit. Embrace the simplicity and richness of herbal living, and watch as it blossoms into a cherished family tradition.

# CONCLUSION

## The Future of Family Wellness with Herbs

As we conclude our exploration of herbal care for children, we look toward a future where families embrace the natural world as a source of healing and wellness. The journey through the chapters of this book has provided a foundation for integrating herbal practices into daily life to nurture the health and well-being of our little ones.

## The Future of Family Wellness with Herbs

The future of family wellness lies in a holistic approach that values the wisdom of nature and the body's innate healing capabilities. Herbs are at the forefront of this approach with their gentle yet powerful properties. As more families discover the benefits of herbal medicine, we can envision a future where natural remedies are a first line of defense against common ailments and preventive care through herbs is the norm rather than the exception.

Integrating herbal practices into family life can transform how we view health care. It encourages a proactive stance on wellness, where families are empowered to take charge of their health using the tools provided by nature. This shift toward natural healing benefits individual families and has broader implications for the health care system and the environment.

# Fostering a Lifelong Connection to Natural Healing

Introducing children to herbal medicine is a gift that can last a lifetime. By teaching them about the healing power of plants, we instill in them a respect for nature and a sense of responsibility for their health. This connection to natural healing can guide them as they grow, influencing their choices and inspiring them to seek holistic solutions.

As parents and caregivers, we nurture this connection, providing a safe and supportive environment for our children to learn and explore. By sharing our experiences with herbs, involving them in growing and using medicinal plants, and encouraging their curiosity, we can help them develop a deep and lasting bond with the natural world.

In conclusion, the journey into herbal care for children is a journey into the heart of nature itself. It's a path that offers health and healing and a deeper understanding of the interconnectedness of all life. As we move forward, let us embrace the future of family wellness with herbs, fostering a lifelong connection to natural healing that will sustain and enrich our children's lives for generations to come.

# APPENDICES

In our journey through the world of herbal care for children, it's essential to navigate with enthusiasm and caution. The appendices provide important safety information and a glossary of kid-friendly herbs to ensure that your experience with natural remedies is both enjoyable and safe.

## Safety Precautions and Contraindications

Before incorporating herbs into your child's wellness routine, there are several safety precautions to keep in mind:

- **Consult with a Healthcare Professional:** Consult with a pediatrician, herbalist, or healthcare provider before giving your child any new herb, especially if they have existing health conditions or are taking medications.

- **Start with Small Doses:** Children's bodies are more sensitive, so begin with smaller doses and observe their reactions.

- **Choose Age-Appropriate Remedies:** Some herbs are unsuitable for infants or young children. Ensure that your herbs are appropriate for your child's age group.

- **Be Aware of Allergies:** Watch for any signs of allergic reactions when introducing new herbs to your child. Symptoms can include skin rashes, itching, or difficulty breathing.

- **Avoid Certain Herbs:** Some herbs, such as ephedra, comfrey, and pennyroyal, should be avoided in children due to potential toxicity or adverse effects.

## Glossary of Kid-Friendly Herbs and Their Uses

Here is a selection of gentle, kid-friendly herbs and their common uses:

- **Chamomile (Matricaria recutita):** Soothes digestion, aids sleep, and calms nerves.
- **Lemon Balm (Melissa officinalis):** Eases anxiety, promotes relaxation, and supports cognitive function.
- **Echinacea (Echinacea spp.):** Boosts the immune system and helps fight colds and flu.
- **Calendula (Calendula officinalis):** Heals skin irritations, minor cuts, and scrapes.
- **Peppermint (Mentha piperita):** Relieves nausea, improves digestion, and freshens breath.
- **Elderberry (Sambucus nigra):** Provides immune support and alleviates cold and flu symptoms.
- **Lavender (Lavandula angustifolia):** Promotes relaxation, aids sleep, and soothes skin irritations.

The appendices serve as a valuable resource for ensuring the safe and effective use of herbal remedies in children. By adhering to safety precautions and familiarizing yourself with the properties of kid-friendly herbs, you can confidently integrate natural healing practices into your family's life. Remember, the journey into herbal care is one of exploration and learning, so continue to seek knowledge and guidance as you nurture your little ones with the gentle power of plants.

# SOURCES

https://www.birthsongbotanicals.com/blogs/birth-song-blog/benefits-using-herbal-remedies-for-children

https://theherbalacademy.com/choosing-safe-herbs-for-your-kids/

https://www.herbsociety.org/hsa-learn/intro-to-herbs/hsa-gardening-for-kids/great-herbs-for-kids.html

https://wholisticmatters.com/healthy-children-herbal-support-for-pediatric-patients/

https://seewhatgrows.org/helpful-herbs-grow-gardening-tips-kids/

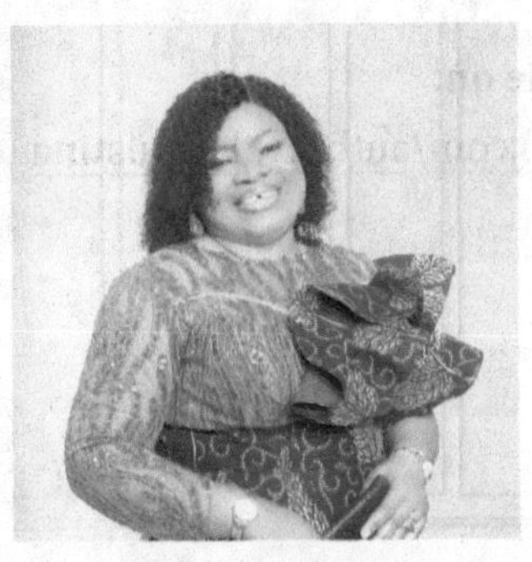

# About the Author

Glorioustina Essia is a multifaceted professional whose expertise traverses the realms of technology, artificial intelligence, literature, and natural health. As a driving force in artificial intelligence, particularly in prompt engineering, she has established herself as a pioneer. Her proficiency extends to project management, network marketing, website development, and copywriting, showcasing a unique blend of technical understanding and creative flair.

A prolific author and publisher, Glorioustina's literary works span multiple genres, captivating a diverse audience with her narrative skill and inspiring a new generation of writers to unlock their creative potential. Her passion for storytelling matches her commitment to exploring and advocating for holistic health practices. Renowned in herbal medicine, she dedicates her life to studying and promoting natural health.

Glorioustina Essia's professional and personal journey is characterized by an unwavering dedication to her core strengths and a ceaseless pursuit of knowledge. Her zeal and expertise embody the limitless possibilities that arise from a commitment to innovation, quality, and a deep-seated passion for understanding the future of technology and the ancient wisdom of herbal medicine. Glorioustina is a testament to the power of interdisciplinary knowledge and its impact in a world where technology, literature, and natural health converge.

**You can connect with me on:**

🌐 https://www.amazon.com/author/glorioustina

# Also by Glorioustina Essia

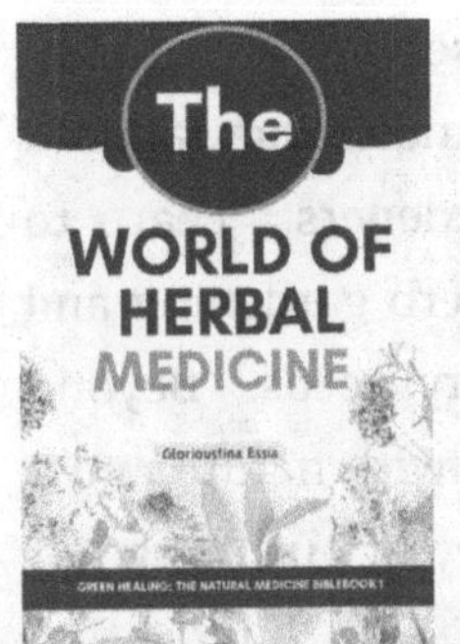

**The World of Herbal Medicine**

In an era where the rush of modern medicine often overshadows the pursuit of holistic health, the timeless wisdom of herbal remedies remains largely untapped. Do you find yourself seeking a more natural approach to health and wellness yet still determining where to begin or how to integrate these practices with modern healthcare?

Embark on a transformative journey with Book 1 of "Green Healing: The Natural Medicine Bible": "The World of Herbal Medicine." This enlightening volume takes you through the ancient pathways to the modern integration of herbal healing. Discover herbal medicine's rich history and evolution across different cultures, including the profound insights of Traditional Chinese Medicine, Ayurveda, and indigenous practices. Unravel how herbalism has evolved through historical epochs and how it beautifully intersects with modern medical practices today.

**Embrace the journey to holistic health – add this captivating volume to your collection and begin exploring the world of herbal medicine today!**

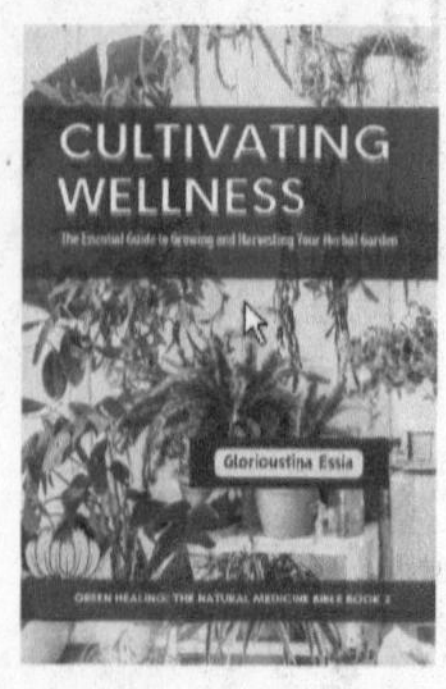

### Cultivating Wellness

This guide is your gateway to mastering the art of herb gardening, offering practical advice for cultivating various medicinal and culinary herbs. From sustainable techniques to harvesting and preservation methods, each chapter brims with expert knowledge tailored to beginners and experienced gardeners. Learn to navigate common challenges in herb gardening and create specialized gardens for your health and culinary needs. Beyond gardening tips, this book inspires a deeper connection with nature and a commitment to a holistic lifestyle. Embrace the journey of nurturing not just a garden but a healthier, more harmonious way of life with "Cultivating Wellness."

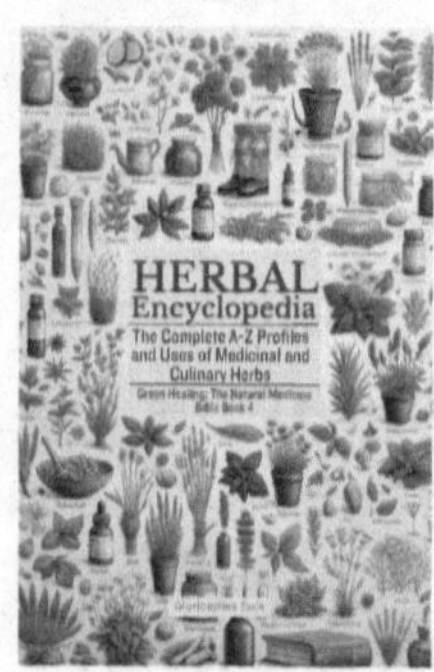

### Herbal Encyclopedia

Embark on a journey through nature's apothecary with "Herbal Encyclopedia: The Complete A-Z Profiles and Uses of Medicinal and Culinary Herbs." This guide unravels the secrets of herbs, from age-old medicinal uses to enhancing culinary delights. Each page introduces you to a new herb, revealing its history, health benefits, and how it can be incorporated into your daily life. Whether you're a budding herbalist or a seasoned enthusiast, this encyclopedia offers easy-to-understand profiles, practical tips, and a connection to the ancient art of herbal healing.

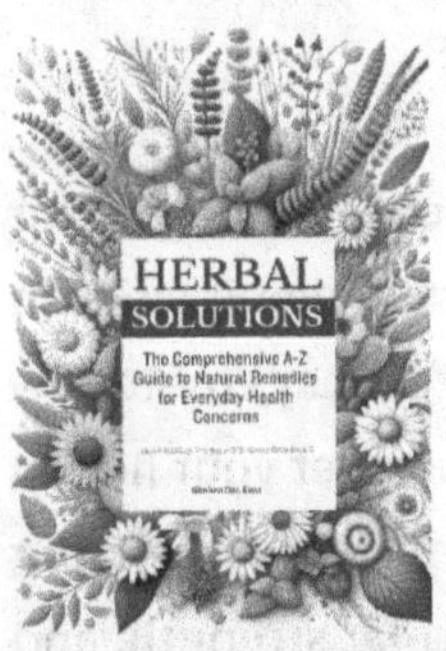

### Herbal Solutions

Discover the secrets to natural wellness with "Herbal Solutions: The Comprehensive A-Z Guide to Natural Remedies for Everyday Health Concerns." This essential resource offers easy-to-access, alphabetical listings of natural remedies for a wide range of common health issues. From herbal solutions to holistic approaches, each entry provides practical, safe, and effective ways to enhance your health naturally. Perfect for those seeking alternative options or complementing traditional medicine, this guide empowers you with the knowledge to take control of your well-being.

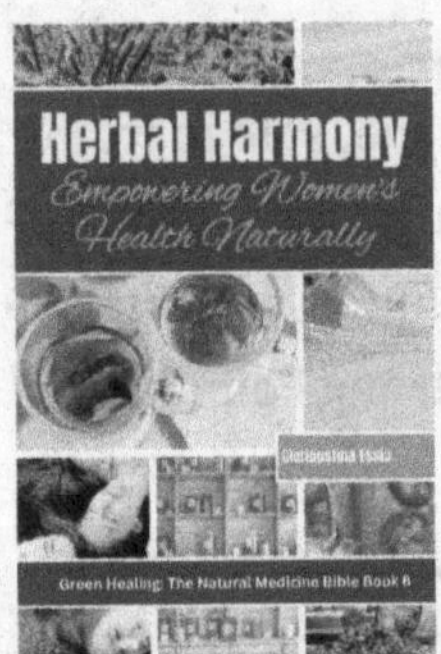

### Herbal Harmony

**Discover the natural path to women's wellness.**

This essential guide illuminates the power of herbs to ease menstrual discomfort, support pregnancy and menopause, and enhance beauty—holistically and safely. From alleviating PMS symptoms to managing menopause gracefully and nurturing your natural beauty, each page is packed with practical advice, effective recipes, and empowering knowledge. Tailored for women at every stage of life, 'Herbal Harmony' offers a treasure trove of herbal remedies that align with your body's natural rhythms.

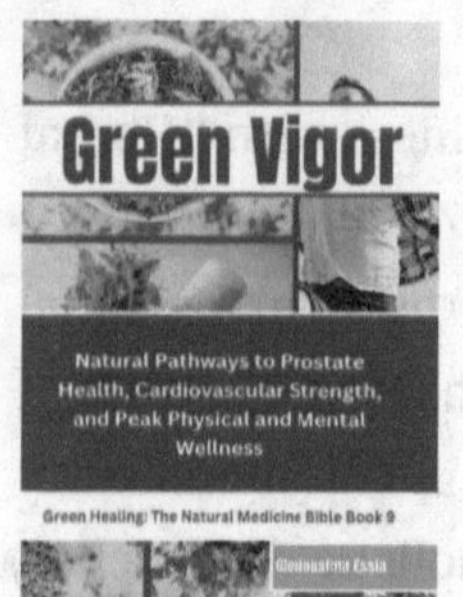

**Green Vigor**

A Man's Guide to Herbal Medicine

Whether you're facing the challenges of aging or simply seeking to optimize your well-being, 'Green Vigor' offers a wealth of knowledge, easy-to-follow recipes, and holistic strategies to empower your health journey. It deepens into natural remedies supporting prostate health, boosting cardiovascular strength, and elevating mental wellness. From ancient herbal wisdom to practical modern applications, discover how to harness nature's bounty to improve your health, reduce stress, and enhance vitality.

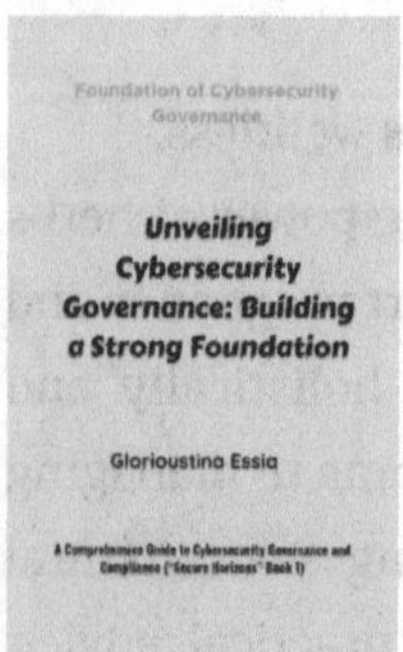

**Unveiling Cybersecurity Governance**

In the ever-expanding digital landscape, safeguarding sensitive information and maintaining robust cyberse-curity practices have become paramount. "Unveiling Cybersecurity Governance: Building a Strong Foundation" is a comprehensive guide that delves into cybersecurity governance's core principles and components, equipping readers with the knowledge and tools to establish a secure digital environment.

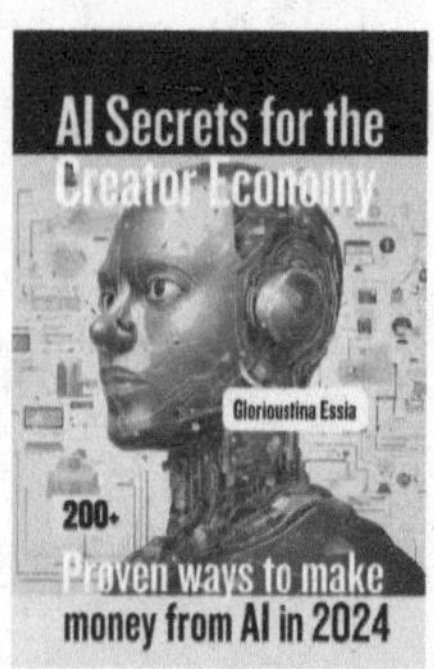

**AI Secrets for the Creator Economy: 200+ Proven ways to make money from AI in 2024**

In a world driven by innovation and transformation, the Creator Economy emerges as a powerful force, with Artificial Intelligence (AI) at its beating heart. This book, "AI Secrets for the Creator Economy: 200+ Proven Ways to Make Money from AI in 2024 and Beyond," is more than just a book; it's your key to unlocking the incredible synergy between AI and creativity, opening the door to a wealth of opportunities for those who are willing to seize them.

www.ingramcontent.com/pod-product-compliance
Lightning Source LLC
Chambersburg PA
CBHW012313240726
48656CB00008B/2666